Antimicrobial Prescribing for General Dental Practitioners

EDITOR: NIKOLAUS O PALMER
BDS MFGDP(UK) PhD FDS RCSEng FFGDP(UK)

FGDP (UK)
PROMOTING EXCELLENCE IN DENTISTRY

Published by
Faculty of General Dental Practice (UK)
The Royal College of Surgeons of England
35-43 Lincoln's Inn Fields
London WC2A 3PE

Tel: 020 7869 6754
Fax: 020 7869 6765
Email: fgdp@rcseng.ac.uk
Website: www.fgdp.org.uk

Registered Charity No. 212808

Antimicrobial Prescribing for General Dental Practitioners

EDITOR: NIKOLAUS O PALMER
BDS MFGDP(UK) PhD FDS RCSEng FFGDP(UK)

ISBN-10: 0-9543451-7-7
ISBN-13: 978-0-9543451-7-4

First edition published 2000 (original title Adult Antimicrobial Prescribing in Primary Dental Care for General Dental Practitioners)
Second edition published 2012

Cover images are reproduced on the cover of this book by kind permission of Professor Wil Colter and Nikolaus O Palmer.

Editorial production: Dave O'Malley, FGDP(UK)
Artworker: Paul Woodcock, FGDP(UK)
Print management: Henry Ling

CONTENTS

CONTENTS

FOREWORD

The FGDP(UK) has declared a commitment to improving the standards of patient care. Through its standards and evidence-based guidelines it aims to help the profession to achieve this goal.

With the increasing problems of antimicrobial resistance, this book provides evidence-based guidance for prudent prescribing and antimicrobial stewardship in the primary care setting.

The purpose of this guidance is not to replace the British National Formulary (BNF) but to provide advice on antimicrobial prescribing; it is not intended to be limiting or restrictive but to be useful in the decision-making process and to be an aid to effective treatment planning and patient care. We believe that this book will prove valuable to general dental practitioners.

Russ Ladwa

Russ Ladwa
Dean , FGDP(UK)

AUTHORS

Dr N O A Palmer

BDS MFGDP(UK) PhD FDS RCSEng FFGDP(UK)

General Dental Practitioner, Crosby, Liverpool

Research Associate, Mersey Deanery, Liverpool

Dr L Longman

BSc, BDS, FDS RCSEd, PhD

Senior Clinical Lecturer and Honorary Consultant in Special Care Dentistry, University of Liverpool

Ms C Randall

BPharm MRPharmS

Senior Medicines Information Pharmacist, North West Medicines Information Centre and National Dental Medicines Information Service, Liverpool

Dr C L Pankhurst

PhD, MSc, BDS, MRCPath, BSc

Specialist in Oral Microbiology

ACKNOWLEDGEMENTS

The authors would like to express their thanks to the following organisations for their comments on drafts of this document.

Association of Dental Implantology UK
The British Dental Association Health and Science Committee
The British Society for Antimicrobial Chemotherapy
The British Society for General Dental Surgery
The British Society for Oral Medicine
The British Society for Paediatric Dentistry
The British Society of Periodontology
Committee of Postgraduate Dental Deans and Directors
The Dental Academy, Portsmouth
The Dental Professionals Association
Scottish Dental Clinical Effectiveness Programme

We would also like to thank the following for their work in preparing this document for publication. Their contributions have been invaluable.

Gareth Kingston
Bill Norris
Dave O'Malley
Justine Wallis
Laura Wiles
Paul Woodcock

1 INTRODUCTION

This guide has been written to help dental practitioners with the prescribing of antimicrobial agents in the primary care dental setting. The guidance given is intended to complement, and not replace, the British National Formulary (BNF).

Registered dentists can legally prescribe from the whole of the BNF, but dentists treating NHS patients are restricted to prescribing antimicrobials included on the Secretary of State's list published in the BNF.[1] Dentists should not prescribe drugs other than to meet the identified dental needs of patients. They must make an appropriate assessment of the patient's condition, prescribe within their experience and competence, and keep accurate records of the treatment.[2]

The aims of these guidelines are to rationalise and improve the standards of antimicrobial prescribing in primary dental care.

This guidance is based on scientific literature and reflects an assessment of the evidence where available. Where the evidence is not available, the authors have relied on wide consultation from specialist groups to obtain a consensus on best clinical practice. The guidance is appropriate for all dental patients, including adults, children and those with special needs who would normally be treated in the primary care setting.

References

1. Joint Formulary Committee. British National Formulary. BNF 63 ed. London: British Medical Association and Royal Pharmaceutical Society of Great Britain; 2012. The reader is reminded that the BNF is constantly revised; for the latest guidelines please consult the current edition at www.BNF.org

2. General Dental Council. Responsible Prescribing. London: GDC; 2008.

2 PRESCRIPTION WRITING

Adapted from the BNF[1] with the kind permission of the Royal Pharmaceutical Society of Great Britain.

Prescriptions should be written legibly in ink or otherwise so as to be indelible, should be dated, should state the full name and address of the patient, and should be signed in ink by the prescriber.

The age and the date of birth of the patient should preferably be stated, and it is a legal requirement in the case of prescription-only medicines to state the age of children under 12 years.

The following should be noted:

a. The unnecessary use of decimal points should be avoided, eg. 3mg, not 3.0mg.
Quantities of one gram or more should be written as 1g, etc.
Quantities of less than one gram should be written in milligrams, eg. 500mg, not 0.5g.
Quantities of less than one milligram should be written in micrograms, eg. 100 micrograms, not 0.1mg.
When decimals are unavoidable, a zero should be written in front of the decimal point where there is no other figure, eg. 0.5ml, not .5ml.
Use of the decimal point is acceptable to express a range, eg. 0.5 to 1g.

b. 'Micrograms' and 'nanograms' should **not** be abbreviated. Similarly 'units' should **not** be abbreviated.

c. The term 'millilitre' (ml or mL) is used in medicine and pharmacy, and cubic centimetre, cc, or cm^3 should not be used.

d. Dose and dose frequency should be stated; in the case of preparations to be taken 'as required,' a **minimum dose interval** should be specified.

e. The names of drugs and preparations should be written clearly and **not** abbreviated, using approved titles **only**.

f. The quantity to be supplied may be stated by indicating the number of days of treatment required in the box provided on NHS forms. In most cases the exact amount will be supplied. This does not apply to items directed to be used as required – if the dose and frequency are not given, then the quantity to be supplied needs to be stated.
When several items are ordered on one form, the box can be marked with the number of days of treatment, provided that the quantity is added for any item for which the amount cannot be calculated.

g. Although directions should preferably be in **English without abbreviation**, it is recognised that some Latin abbreviations are used.

h. Dental practitioners may prescribe unlicensed medicines (ie. those without marketing authorisation), medicines used 'off-label' (ie. those being used for an indication not included in the marketing authorisation), or withdrawn medicines. The prescriber should inform the patient or the patient's carer that the product does not have a marketing authorisation.

Never prescribe a drug unless there is a good clinical indication

Make prescriptions clear

Use approved names

Always make the source of the prescription clear

Always record prescription details in the clinical notes

Avoid prescribing during pregnancy whenever possible

Avoid abbreviations – give the name of the drug in full

References

1. Joint Formulary Committee. British National Formulary. BNF 63 ed. London: British Medical Association and Royal Pharmaceutical Society of Great Britain; 2012. The reader is reminded that the BNF is constantly revised; for the latest guidelines please consult the current edition at www.BNF.org

3 PRESCRIBING ANTIMICROBIALS

Dentists working in primary care prescribe antimicrobials to manage oral and dental infections. The benefits of prescribing antimicrobials are however limited by a number of problems associated with their use eg. side effects, allergic reactions, toxicity and the development of resistant strains of microbes.[1]

Within the last few decades antimicrobial resistance has become a worldwide problem and constitutes a major threat to public health.[2] The indiscriminate prescribing of antimicrobials by health care professionals is targeted as a major factor to be addressed. Dentists working in NHS primary care prescribe nearly 10% of all the oral antimicrobials prescribed in primary care in England.[3] There is increasing evidence of the inappropriate use of antimicrobials in dentistry and this may contribute to the problem of antimicrobial resistance.[4-7] The use of antimicrobials leads to selection and dominance of resistant micro-organisms; they can also increase the incidence of resistance through the exchange of genetic material, so that resistant genes can spread between bacterial populations.

Dentists should be aware that serious drug interactions can occur with antimicrobial agents when other drugs are taken concomitantly (eg. miconazole/fluconazole and warfarin, erythromycin and simvastatin). Dentists should also be aware that prescribing for the elderly, expectant and nursing mothers, patients that have comorbidities (eg. renal or liver impairment) may require modification. Dentists are advised to always check the BNF or other authoritative source, such as the *Electronic Medicines Compendium*.[8]

Information on any aspect of drug therapy can be obtained from the UK Medicines Information service by phoning your regional Medicines Information (MI) centre; numbers can be found inside the front cover of the British National Formulary. The regional MI centre in the North West (NWMIC) provides a specialist service on drug use in dentistry and can be contacted on

0151 794 8206. For further information about the NWMIC and to access documents related to dentistry, visit www.ukmi.nhs.uk/activities/specialistServices

3.1 Indications for prescribing antimicrobials

Antimicrobial prescribing in primary care is only indicated:

- As an **adjunct** to the management of acute or chronic infection.
- For the definitive management of active infective disease, eg. necrotising ulcerative gingivitis.
- Where definitive treatment has to be delayed due to referral to specialist services. Examples would include: an inability to establish drainage in an uncooperative patient who requires sedation or general anaesthesia for treatment; or a patient who needs to be treated in a hospital environment due to comorbidities.

There is no indication for the prescribing of antimicrobials for acute pulpitis, where definitive treatment of the cause along with analgesics is more appropriate.[9,10]

References

1. Finch RG. Adverse reactions to antibiotics. In: Greenwood D, editor. Antimicrobial chemotherapy, 4th ed. Oxford: Oxford University Press; 2000. p. 200-11.

2. House of Lords Select Committee on Science and Technology, Seventh Report. Resistance to antibiotics and other antimicrobial agents. London: HMSO; 1998.

3. The NHS Information Centre. Prescribing by dentists 2010: England. Available at: www.ic.nhs.uk/statistics-and-data-collections/primary-care/dentistry/prescribing-by-dentists-2010-england. Accessed: September 2011.

4. Palmer NA, Pealing R, Ireland RS, Martin MV. A study of prophylactic antibiotic prescribing in National Health Service general dental practice in England. Br Dent J 2000;189(1):43-6.

5. Palmer NA, Pealing R, Ireland RS, Martin MV. A study of therapeutic antibiotic prescribing in National Health Service general dental practice in England. Br Dent J 2000;188(10):554-8.

6. Harte H, Palmer NO, Martin MV. An investigation of therapeutic antibiotic prescribing for children referred for dental general anaesthesia in three community National Health Service trusts. Br Dent J 2005;198(4):227-31,

7. Tulip DE, Palmer NO. A retrospective investigation of the clinical management of patients attending an out of hours dental clinic in Merseyside under the new NHS dental contract. Br Dent J 2008;205(12):659-64,

8. The Electronic Medicines Compendium. http://www.medicines.org.uk/emc

9. Brennan MT, Runyon MS, Batts JJ, Fox PC, Kent ML, Cox TL, et al. Odontogenic signs and symptoms as predictors of odontogenic infection: a clinical trial. J Am Dent Assoc 2006;137(1):62-6.

10. Nagle D, Reader A, Beck M, Weaver J. Effect of systemic penicillin on pain in untreated irreversible pulpitis. Oral Surg Oral Med Oral Pathol Oral Radiol Endod 2000;90(5):636-40.

4 ACUTE DENTO-ALVEOLAR INFECTIONS

Early recognition and management of dento-alveolar infections is critical because patients (particularly children and immunocompromised patients) can become systemically ill within a short time.[1,2] If untreated, local infections can spread, giving rise to serious life-threatening sequelae, eg. Ludwig's angina.

The initial assessment of the patient should include the following:

- Taking a comprehensive medical and dental history.[3]
- Checking for the presence of fever, malaise, fatigue, dizziness or other debility.
- Measuring the pulse and temperature (normal axillary temperature is 36.3°C - 37°C).
- Defining the nature, location and extent of the swelling.
- Identifying the cause of the infection.

Following this assessment, the clinician should decide whether treatment can be provided in primary care or whether a referral is necessary; for example, if there is/are:

- Signs of septicaemia such as grossly elevated temperature (ie. above 39.5°C), lethargy, tachycardia.
- Spreading cellulitis.
- Swellings that may compromise the airway, or cause difficulty in swallowing or closure of the eye.
- Dehydration.
- Significant trismus associated with a dental infection.
- Failure to respond to previous treatment.
- An uncooperative patient.

4.1 Management of acute dento-alveolar infections

- The majority of uncomplicated infected swellings of dental origin can be successfully treated by removal of the source of the infection by drainage of the associated abscess, removal of infected pulp contents or by extraction of the tooth.[4]
- Antimicrobials are only indicated as an adjunct to definitive treatment where there is an elevated temperature, evidence of systemic spread and local lymph gland involvement.[4,5]
- Ensure that fluid balance is maintained.
- Follow-up of the patient 2-3 days after drainage and removal of the cause. If there is resolution of the infection and the temperature is normal, stop antimicrobials[6].
- Failure of resolution is usually caused by failure to establish adequate drainage, poor host resistance, poor patient compliance or the wrong diagnosis.[6] **Re-establish drainage or refer for specialist advice.**

The algorithm for management of acute dento-alveolar infections is shown in *Fig 1*.

Management of acute dento-alveolar infections

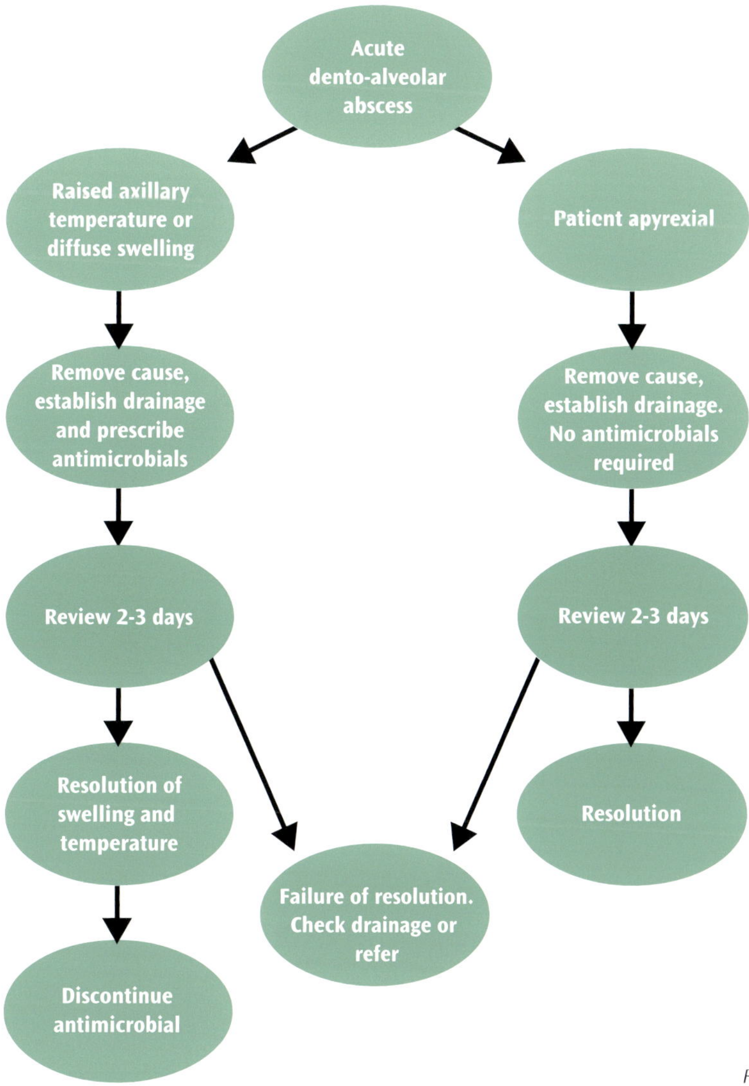

Fig 1

4.2 Choice of antimicrobial

First choice antimicrobial

The first choice is a penicillin, such as amoxicillin, which has been shown to be effective, particularly in the management of infections in children.[7] Phenoxymethylpenicillin is equally effective but less reliably absorbed and needs to be taken four times daily on an empty stomach.

AMOXICILLIN

Adults

Amoxicillin 250mg three times daily for up to five days[6]

Children

- Under 12 months old: 62.5mg three times daily for up to five days
- 1-5 years old: 125mg three times daily for up to five days
- 6-12 years old: 250mg three times daily for up to five days

Available on prescription as:

- Amoxicillin capsules 250mg
- Amoxicillin oral suspension (sugar-free) 125mg/5mL
- Amoxicillin oral suspension (sugar-free) 250mg/5mL

Second choice antimicrobial

The second choice antimicrobial is metronidazole which can also be used:

- as first-line treatment for patients who are allergic to penicillin; or
- as first-line treatment for patients who have had a recent course of penicillin for another infection; or
- as an adjunct to amoxicillin in severe spreading infections; or
- if a predominantly anaerobic infection is suspected or microbiologically proven.

METRONIDAZOLE

Adults

Metronidazole 200mg three times daily for three days[8]

Children

- 1-3 years: 50mg three times daily for three days
- 3-7 years: 100mg twice daily for three days
- 7-10 years: 100mg three times daily for three days
- Over 10 years: 200mg three times daily for three days

Available on prescription as:

- Metronidazole tablets 200mg
- Metronidazole oral suspension 200mg/5ml

Third choice antimicrobial

The third choice antimicrobial is a macrolide, eg. azithromycin, clarithromycin or erythromycin. These can be used as an alternative to a penicillin. Azithromycin and clarithromycin are better tolerated than erythromycin, which causes nausea, vomiting and diarrhoea in some patients, and many organisms are resistant to it.

CLARITHROMYCIN

Adults

Clarithromycin 250mg twice daily for up to five days

continued...

Children

1 month-12 years

- Bodyweight under 8kg: 7.5mg/kg twice daily
- Bodyweight 8-11kg: 62.5mg twice daily
- Bodyweight 12-19kg: 125mg twice daily
- Bodyweight 20-29kg: 187.5mg twice daily
- Bodyweight 30-40kg: 250mg twice daily

12–18 years

- 250mg twice daily for up to 5 days

Available on prescription as:

- Clarithromycin tablets 250mg
- Clarithromycin oral suspension 125mg/5ml
- Clarithromycin oral suspension 250mg/5ml

OR

AZITHROMYCIN

Adults

Azithromycin 500mg once daily for 2-3 days

Children

- 6 months-3 years: 10mg/kg once a day for 2-3 days
- 3-7 years: 200mg once a day for 2-3 days

continued...

- 8-11 years: 300mg once a day for 2-3 days
- 12-14 years: 400mg once a day for 2-3 days
- Over 14 years: 500mg once a day for 2-3 days

Available on prescription as:

- Azithromycin capsules 250mg
- Azithromycin tablets 250mg
- Azithromycin tablets 500mg
- Azithromycin oral suspension 200mg/5ml

The prescribing of clindamycin, cephalosporins or co-amoxiclav offers no advantage over a penicillin, metronidazole or a macrolide and is not recommended for the routine management of dento-alveolar infections.

The inappropriate use of clindamycin, cephalosporins or co-amoxiclav will contribute to the development of resistance to these drugs and can lead to the development of *Clostridium difficile* infection.

The use of antibiotics other than recommended in this guidance should only be at the direction of a specialist.

References

1. Dodson TB, Perrott DH, Kaban LB. Pediatric maxillofacial infections: a retrospective study of 113 patients. J Oral Maxillofac Surg 1989;47(4):327-30.

2. Sandor GK, Low DE, Judd PL, Davidson RJ. Antimicrobial treatment options in the management of odontogenic infections. J Can Dent Assoc 1998;64(7):508-14.

3. Faculty of General Dental Practice (UK). Clinical examination and record-keeping: good practice guidelines, 2nd ed. London: Faculty of General Dental Practice (UK); 2009.

4. Matthews DC, Sutherland S, Basrani B. Emergency management of acute apical abscesses in the permanent dentition: a systematic review of the literature. J Can Dent Assoc 2003;69(10):660.

5. Matthews D, Sutherland S. Clinical practice guidelines on emergency management of acute apical periodontitis and acute apical abscess. Evid Based Dent 2004;5:7-11.

6. Martin MV, Longman LP, Hill JB, Hardy P. Acute dento-alveolar infections: an investigation of the duration of antibiotic therapy. Br Dent J 1997;183(4):135-7.

7. Paterson SA, Curzon ME. The effect of amoxycillin versus penicillin V in the treatment of acutely abscessed primary teeth. Br Dent J 1993;174(12):443-9.

8. Joint Formulary Committee. British National Formulary. BNF 63 ed. London: British Medical Association and Royal Pharmaceutical Society of Great Britain; 2012. The reader is reminded that the BNF is constantly revised; for the latest guidelines please consult the current edition at www.BNF.org.

5 CHRONIC DENTO-ALVEOLAR INFECTIONS

Chronic dento-alveolar infections can occur in association with decayed or restored teeth. They commonly present as a minor, well localised abscess, sometimes with a discharging sinus and rarely require antimicrobial therapy unless:

- There is an acute flare-up and there is evidence of gross local spread; or
- There is systemic involvement shown by an elevated temperature or malaise.

The principles of treatment are:

- Removal of the cause.
- Drainage of the infection.

The algorithm for managing chronic dento-alveolar infections is shown in *Fig 2*. Antimicrobial choice is as for acute dento-alveolar infections (see Chapter 4).

Long-standing chronic infections which do not respond to simple treatment (eg. osteomyelitis) should be referred to a consultant specialist.

Management of chronic dento-alveolar infections

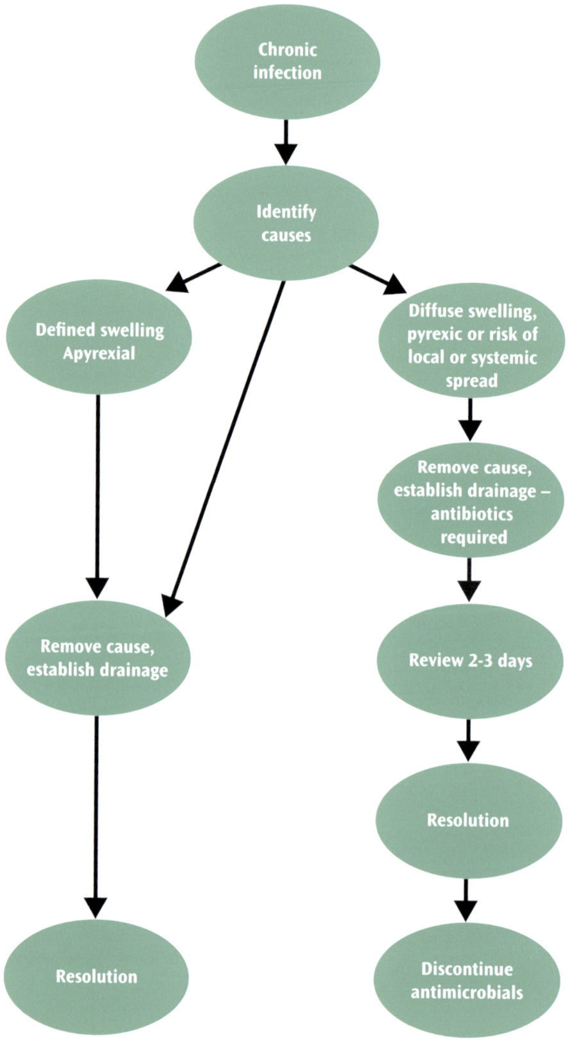

Fig 2

6 PERIODONTAL DISEASE

6.1 Gingivitis

There are no indications for the prescribing of systemic antimicrobials for the management of gingivitis.

6.2 Periodontal abscess

For management options, see Chapter 4.1: Management of acute dento-alveolar infections.

The majority of uncomplicated infected swellings of periodontal origin can be successfully treated by removing the source of the infection. This can be achieved by drainage of the associated abscess by root surface debridement via the pocket or by extraction of the tooth.[1,2]

Antimicrobials are only indicated as an adjunct to definitive treatment where there is an elevated temperature, evidence of systemic spread and local lymph gland involvement.[1,2]

6.3 Necrotising ulcerative gingivitis

As an adjunct to local measures (scaling and oral hygiene instruction) the antimicrobial of choice is metronidazole due to the anaerobic nature of the infection.[3-5]

METRONIDAZOLE

Adults

Metronidazole 200mg three times daily for three days[5]

Children

- 1-3 years: 50mg three times daily for three days
- 3-7 years: 100mg twice daily for three days
- 7-10 years: 100mg three times daily for three days
- Over 10 years: 200mg three times daily for three days

Available on prescription as:

- Metronidazole tablets 200mg
- Metronidazole oral suspension 200mg/5ml

For patients who cannot take metronidazole (eg. because of alcohol dependency, pregnancy, drug interactions) amoxicillin is the drug of choice.

AMOXICILLIN

Adults

Amoxicillin 250mg three times daily for up to five days[6]

Children

- Under 12 months old: 62.5mg three times daily for up to five days
- 1-5 years old: 125mg three times daily for up to five days
- 6-12 years old: 250mg three times daily for up to five days

continued...

Available on prescription as:

- Amoxicillin capsules 250mg
- Amoxicillin oral suspension (sugar-free) 125mg/5mL
- Amoxicillin oral suspension (sugar-free) 250mg/5mL

6.4 Aggressive periodontitis

Following the diagnosis of aggressive periodontitis, the practitioner should consider referral to a specialist.

In cases of aggressive periodontitis, systematic reviews demonstrate that adjunctive systemic antimicrobials can result in greater probing depth reductions and gains in clinical attachment compared to just root surface debridement, but only in the short term.[7-11]

If systemic antibiotics are used as part of periodontal therapy, they should be used only as an adjunct to thorough and effective mechanical debridement.

There is no direct evidence to recommend a specific protocol for adjunctive systemic antibiotics with root surface debridement.[8]

6.5 Chronic periodontitis

In the majority of patients with chronic periodontitis, the prescribing of systemic antimicrobials as an adjunct to subgingival mechanical debridement is not indicated.[7,8]

The long-term benefits of prescribing systemic antimicrobials in patients with severe chronic periodontitis as an adjunct to local measures have not been proven. Clinicians therefore need to weigh any short-term benefits of systemic antimicrobial treatment against the potential for adverse effects at both the individual and general population level.

In patients with severe or progressing forms of periodontitis that have responded poorly to thorough and effective mechanical debridement and excellent patient oral hygiene, adjunctive antimicrobials may improve outcomes. There is, however, no evidence of the superiority of one antibiotic protocol over another for their use.[7] Practitioners should consider referring these unresponsive chronic periodontitis cases to a specialist.

Sub-antimicrobial dose doxycycline (Periostat®), which reduces the elevated collagenase activity present in chronic periodontitis, has been shown to enhance pocket depth reductions in patients with chronic periodontitis, but only when used as an adjunct to thorough root surface debridement and excellent home care by the patient.[12]

DOXYCYCLINE

Adults

Doxycycline 20mg twice daily for three months

Children

Not indicated

Available on prescription as Doxycycline tablets, 20mg (Periostat®)

The local use of antimicrobials has been shown to be of no value.[13,14]

References

1. Matthews DC, Sutherland S, Basrani B. Emergency management of acute apical abscesses in the permanent dentition: a systematic review of the literature. J Can Dent Assoc 2003;69(10):660.

2. Matthews D, Sutherland S. Clinical practice guidelines on emergency management of acute apical periodontitis and acute apical abscess. Evid Based Dent 2004;5:7-11.

3. Johnson BD, Engel D. Acute necrotizing ulcerative gingivitis. A review of diagnosis, etiology and treatment. J Periodontol 1986;57(3):141-50.

4. Shinn DL. Metronidazole in acute ulcerative gingivitis. Lancet 1962;1:1191.

5. Duckworth R, Waterhouse JP, Britton DE, Nuki K, Sheiham A, Winter R, et al. Acute ulcerative gingivitis. A double-blind controlled clinical trial of metronidazole. Br Dent J 1966;120(12):599-602.

6. Martin MV, Longman LP, Hill JB, Hardy P. Acute dento-alveolar infections: an investigation of the duration of antibiotic therapy. Br Dent J 1997;183(4):135-7.

7. Herrera D, Alonso B, Leon R, Roldan S, Sanz M. Antimicrobial therapy in periodontitis: the use of systemic antimicrobials against the subgingival biofilm. J Clin Periodontol 2008;35(8 Suppl):45-66.

8. Herrera D, Sanz M, Jepsen S, Needleman I, Roldan S. A systematic review on the effect of systemic antimicrobials as an adjunct to scaling and root planing in periodontitis patients. J Clin Periodontol 2002;29(3 Suppl):136-59.

9. Guerrero A, Griffiths GS, Nibali L, Suvan J, Moles DR, Laurell L, et al. Adjunctive benefits of systemic amoxicillin and metronidazole in non-surgical treatment of generalized aggressive periodontitis: a randomized placebo-controlled clinical trial. J Clin Periodontol 2005;32(10):1096-107.

10. Winkel EG, Van Winkelhoff AJ, Timmerman MF, Van der Velden U, Van der Weijden GA. Amoxicillin plus metronidazole in the treatment of adult periodontitis patients. A double-blind placebo-controlled study. J Clin Periodontol 2001;28(4):296-305.

11. Varela VM, Heller D, Silva-Senem MX,Torres MC,Colombo AP, Feres-Filho EJ. Systemic antimicrobials adjunctive to a repeated mechanical and antiseptic therapy for aggressive periodontitis: a 6-month randomized controlled trial. J Periodontol 2011;82(8):1121-30.

12. Preshaw PM, Novak MJ, Mellonig J, Magnusson I, Polson A, Giannobile WV, et al. Modified-release subantimicrobial dose doxycycline enhances scaling and root planing in subjects with periodontal disease. J Periodontol 2008;79(3):440-52.

13. Bonito AJ, Lux L, Lohr KN. Impact of local adjuncts to scaling and root planing in periodontal disease therapy: a systematic review. J Periodontol 2005;76(8):1227-36.

14. Tomasi C, Koutouzis T, Wennstrom JL. Locally delivered doxycycline as an adjunct to mechanical debridement at retreatment of periodontal pockets. J Periodontol 2008;79(3):431-9.

7 PERICORONITIS

The treatment of pericoronitis is by local measures. These include:

- Debridement and irrigation of accessible stagnation areas (abscesses may need incision and drainage).
- Operculectomy.[1]
- Occlusal adjustment to relieve occlusion, or extract opposing tooth if it is traumatising any inflamed pericoronal tissues.[1]
- Extraction of the impacted tooth, if there has been more than one episode, when infection is under control.[2]

Local measures are sufficient unless:[1]

- Temperature is raised.
- There is a spreading infection or severe localised infection or persistent swelling despite local measures.
- Trismus is present.

Metronidazole is the antimicrobial of choice as an adjunct to local measures. Amoxicillin is a suitable alternative where metronidazole is contraindicated.

The algorithm for managing pericoronitis is shown in *Fig 3*.

METRONIDAZOLE

Adults

Metronidazole tablets 200mg three times daily for three days

Children

- 1-3 years: 50mg three times daily for three days
- 3-7 years: 100mg twice daily for three days
- 7-10 years: 100mg three times daily for three days
- Over 10 years: 200mg three times daily for three days

Available on prescription as:

- Metronidazole tablets 200mg
- Metronidazole oral suspension 200mg/5ml

OR

AMOXICILLIN

Adults

Amoxicillin 250mg three times daily for three days

Children

- Under 12 months old: 62.5mg three times daily for up to five days
- 1-5 years old: 125mg three times daily for up to five days
- 6-12 years old: 250mg three times daily for up to five days

Available on prescription as:

- Amoxicillin capsules 250mg
- Amoxicillin oral suspension (sugar-free) 125mg/5ml
- Amoxicillin oral suspension (sugar-free) 250mg/5ml

Management of Pericoronitis

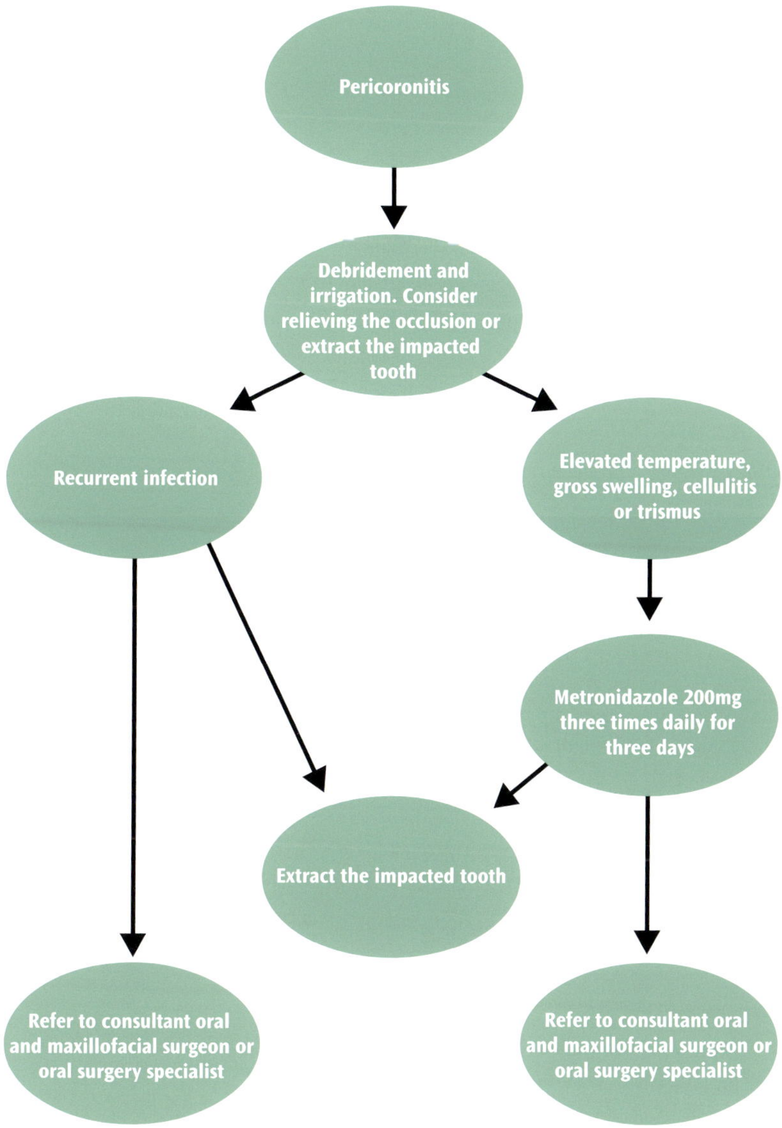

Fig 3

References

1. Faculty of Dental Surgery. National Clinical Guidelines 1997. London: The Royal College of Surgeons of England, 1997 (reviewed 2004).

2. National Institute for Health and Clinical Excellence. Technology Appraisal Guidance 1: Guidance on the extraction of wisdom teeth. London: NICE;2000.

8 MANAGEMENT OF DRY SOCKET

Dry socket or localised osteitis is a recognised complication following tooth extraction, with incidence rates thought to be in the region of 4%. Usually it occurs 3-4 days post-extraction and lasts for up to 10 days.[1-3]

The aetiology is thought to be associated with surgical trauma, localised infection and systemic factors. In the absence of a spreading infection antimicrobials are contraindicated. Management is centred around local measures:[2]

- If necessary, radiograph to exclude a foreign body or root.
- Irrigate with chlorhexidine to remove debris.[2,4]
- Pack the socket with a suitable dressing, eg. Alvogyl®.
- Prescribe analgesics; non-steroidal anti-inflammatory drugs are preferred if they are tolerated and there are no contraindications.[2,4]
- Review the patient.

References

1. Monaco G, Staffolani C, Gatto MR, Checchi L. Antibiotic therapy in impacted third molar surgery. Eur J Oral Sci 1999;107(6):437-41.

2. Noroozi AR, Philbert RF. Modern concepts in understanding and management of the "dry socket" syndrome: comprehensive review of the literature. Oral Surg Oral Med Oral Pathol Oral Radiol Endod 2009;107(1):30-5.

3. Hill M. No benefit from prophylactic antibiotics in third molar surgery. Evid Based Dent 2005;6(1):10.

4. Blum IR. Contemporary views on dry socket (alveolar osteitis): a clinical appraisal of standardization, aetiopathogenesis and management: a critical review. Int J Oral Maxillofac Surg 2002;31(3):309-17.

9 ACUTE SINUSITIS (RHINOSINUSITIS)

Most cases of acute sinusitis are viral and usually follow a cold. Acute sinusitis can be diagnosed by:

- Nasal discharge – should be clear; a thick purulent, coloured discharge (especially green) may indicate a bacterial infection.
- Nasal blockage or congestion – usually bilateral and caused by rhinitis.
- Facial pain – localised over the affected sinus and may be described as pressure. May affect teeth, the upper jaw or eye, side of face or forehead. Pain in the absence of other symptoms is unlikely to be sinusitis.
- Loss of sense of smell.

Most cases of uncomplicated acute sinusitis respond to watchful waiting and measures to relieve symptoms:[1,2]

- Paracetamol or ibuprofen to relieve pain and fever.
- Intranasal decongestant (maximum one week).
- Saline nasal drops or irrigation.
- Warm face packs.
- Adequate fluids and rest.

Antimicrobials are rarely indicted as they offer little benefit for patients with acute sinusitis. They are not justified even if a patient reports symptoms for longer than 7-10 days.

Where the symptoms are more severe or complicated by systemic illness, serious local infection or existing co-morbidities, eg. immunosuppression or significant heart, lung, renal, liver or neuromuscular disease, the patient should be referred to their general medical practitioner or for specialist advice.[1,2]

References

1. National Institute for Health and Clinical Excellence. CG69: Prescribing of antibiotics for self-limiting respiratory tract infections in adults and children in primary care. London: NICE; 2009. Available at: www.nice.org.uk/CG69. Accessed: 24 Mar 2011.

2. PRODIGY (2011) *Sinusitus*. http://www.prodigy.clarity.co.uk/sinusitis. Accessed: Feb 2012.

10 ENDODONTIC THERAPY

The clinical management options for infection of endodontic origin are:

- Root canal therapy.
- Retreatment of existing root canal therapy.
- Periradicular surgery.
- Extraction.

Antimicrobials are **not** indicated in endodontic therapy unless:

- There is evidence of gross local spread of infection (see Chapter 4: Acute dento-alveolar infections).
- There is systemic evidence of infection (eg. pyrexia).
- Drainage cannot be achieved immediately or treatment has to be delayed, eg. referral for periradicular surgery.

Administration of antimicrobials postoperatively does not reduce pain, percussion pain, swelling, or the number of analgesics taken in symptomatic root-filled teeth.[1,2]

References

1. Pickenpaugh L, Reader A, Beck M, Meyers WJ, Peterson LJ. Effect of prophylactic amoxicillin on endodontic flare-up in asymptomatic, necrotic teeth. J Endod 2001;27(1):53-6.

2. Henry M, Reader A, Beck M. Effect of penicillin on postoperative endodontic pain and swelling in symptomatic necrotic teeth. J Endod 2001;27(2):117-23.

11 PROPHYLACTIC ANTIMICROBIALS

Antimicrobial prophylaxis is the prevention of infection by the administration of antimicrobial agents. It remains a contentious issue in all surgical fields and medical specialties. Ideally the administration of antimicrobials should reduce morbidity and mortality. In reality they may cause drug interactions, adverse effects (allergy, toxicity) and reduce colonisation resistance, resulting in infections with resistant micro-organisms.

The medico-legal and ethical issues are highlighted below:

- The at-risk group must be easily identifiable to prevent overuse.
- Prophylaxis must be efficacious and reliable.
- Proof of efficacy must be without question.
- Prophylaxis must not cause more harm than the infection being prevented.
- A bacteraemia has to be the cause of patient disease.
- The antimicrobial is only aimed at the causative pathogen.

11.1 Antimicrobial prophylaxis for healthy patients

Antimicrobials have sometimes been prescribed for healthy patients in the following circumstances.

11.1.1 Minor oral surgery (removal of impacted teeth, roots, peri-radicular surgery)

There is no evidence for the prophylactic use of antimicrobials to prevent postoperative infection as a result of the surgical removal of impacted teeth or roots. Additionally, no difference was found with regard to the prevention of postoperative infection in endodontic surgical procedures.[1] Conversely evidence exists that prophylactic use of antimicrobials has no effect on post operative pain, swelling, infection or wound healing.[2-4]

11.1.2 Reimplantation of teeth

A number of guidelines exist that suggest that the practitioner should consider prescribing antimicrobials when reimplanting an avulsed tooth.[5,6] There is, however, no scientific evidence that antimicrobial use improves the success rate of re-implanted teeth.

11.1.3 Periodontal surgery

There is not enough evidence to support the routine use of prophylactic antimicrobials for the prevention of postoperative infections following periodontal surgery.[7,8]

11.1.4 Endodontic therapy

See Chapter 10: Endodontic therapy.

11.1.5 Placing of implants

Some implant manufacturers have suggested a number of different protocols for antimicrobial prescribing when implants are placed. They have suggested that their use reduces the incidence of postoperative infections, peri-implantitis and postoperative pain. However, this remains a controversial issue, with little good-quality evidence to support the use of routine prophylactic antimicrobials in the placing of implants.

It has been shown that antimicrobials do not provide significant advantages concerning postoperative infections in the presence of good asepsis.[9] However, a meta-analysis including only four randomised controlled trials concluded that there is some evidence suggesting that the following protocol significantly reduces implant failure:[10]

Amoxicillin 2g (4 × 500mg capsules) one hour preoperatively

In the absence of any published scientific evidence with patients who are allergic to penicillins, the following protocol is suggested:

Clindamycin 600mg (4 × 150mg capsules) one hour preoperatively

11.1.6 Oroantral communications and fistulae

Oroantral communications are a well recognised complication of tooth extraction. They may be caused by operative treatment or by the patient not following post-operative instructions. Successful management is dependent on:

- Establishing the cause.
- Primary closure by a suitably competent practitioner if no infection is present.
- Referral if primary closure not possible.
- Prescribing of antimicrobials, as follows:[11]

AMOXICILLIN

Adults

Amoxicillin 250mg three times daily for up to five days

Children

- Under 12 months old: 62.5mg three times daily for up to five days

continued...

- 1-5 years old: 125mg three times daily for up to five days
- 6-12 years old: 250mg three times daily for up to five days

Available on prescription as:

- Amoxicillin capsules 250mg
- Amoxicillin oral suspension (sugar-free) 125mg/5ml
- Amoxicillin oral suspension (sugar-free) 250mg/5ml

OR

DOXYCYCLINE

Adults and children over 12 years

Doxycycline 200mg stat followed by 100mg daily for five days

Doxycycline is contraindicated in children under 12 years

Available on prescription as:

- Doxycycline capsules 100mg
- Doxycycline dispersible tablets 100mg

11.2 Antimicrobial prophylaxis for medically compromised patients

In the past, antimicrobials have been prescribed prophylactically to prevent bacteraemias and metastatic infections as a result of dental treatment. The evidence for bacteraemias associated with dental procedures has been reviewed, specifically in relation to cardiac patients. It has been concluded by the British Society of Antimicrobial Chemotherapy (BSAC) and the National Institute for Health and Clinical Excellence (NICE) that the magnitude and frequency of bacteraemias resulting from normal oral function (eg. chewing, toothbrushing) is greater than that from dental procedures.[12]

11.2.1 Cardiac patients

Prior to the publication of NICE guidelines, patients with acquired or congenital endocardial disease were required to have antimicrobial prophylaxis prior to a number of dental procedures. The NICE guidelines advise that there is no need for antimicrobial prophylaxis for such patients.[13]

11.2.2 Total joint replacements

Bacteraemias as a result of dental procedures have been implicated in infections of total joint replacements. However the evidence is tenuous and unproven, relying on anecdotal case reports.[14] A recent case-control study confirmed that dental treatment was not a risk factor for subsequent total joint infections.[15]

The evidence in relation to dental treatment, associated bacteraemias and metastatic infections reviewed by NICE for cardiac patients[13] is also relevant for total joint replacements. The BSAC found no indication for antimicrobial prophylaxis for dental procedures on patients with total joint replacement.[16]

11.2.3 Miscellaneous prosthetic implants

Patients with cardiac pacemakers, penile, breast or intra-ocular implants and prosthetic vascular grafts have never been considered susceptible to infection from dental bacteraemias.[17,18]

Intravascular access devices, such as central intravenous lines used for total parenteral nutrition or chemotherapy, and catheters for haemodialysis and plasmapheresis, do not require antibiotic cover for dental treatment.[18]

Despite there being no clear evidence,[19] patients receiving renal dialysis are recommended by some renal specialists as requiring antimicrobial prophylaxis. The BSAC recommends that prophylaxis is not required for dental procedures in these patients.[18]

11.2.4 Immunocompromised patients

Immune function may be impaired by a range of conditions, such as leukaemia, immunosuppressive drugs following organ transplantation, lymphomas, anti-cancer chemotherapy, poorly controlled diabetes, and HIV. In all of these patients, infections can be life-threatening. The importance of maintaining good dental care and treating odontogenic infections aggressively in these patients cannot be overemphasised.

There is no clear evidence that these patients are at risk of infections as a result of dental procedures, and therefore the routine use of antimicrobial prophylaxis in this group of patients cannot be supported.[18]

Transplant patients are immunosuppressed by their drug therapy and have been considered to be at risk for local and systemic infection. In the immediate post-transplant period it is best that routine dental treatment is delayed until the patient is in the stable post-transplant phase, usually six months after surgery.

Emergency treatment should be carried out in conjunction with advice from the patient's specialist.

11.2.5 Bisphosphonate-related osteonecrosis of the jaw (BRONJ)

There is no evidence to support the routine use of antimicrobial prophylaxis for patients taking oral bisphosphonates undergoing dental treatment.[20]

11.2.6 Radiotherapy

Patients who have previously been exposed to, or are currently undergoing, radiotherapy to the head and neck may be susceptible to local infection as a result of the diminution of the vascular supply to the irradiated area. This risk increases with time. Careful assessment of patients prior to radiotherapy and maintenance of good oral health is important.

It is important that teeth should not be extracted, where possible, as the risk of osteonecrosis is high.

The efficacy of antimicrobials is questionable due to the poor blood flow and tissue penetration in the irradiated area. Nevertheless, antimicrobial prophylaxis is recommended by some authorities, and if a tooth cannot be saved, advice on management should be sought from a maxillofacial surgeon.[21]

References

1. Lindeboom JA, Frenken JW, Valkenburg P, van den Akker HP. The role of preoperative prophylactic antibiotic administration in periapical endodontic surgery: a randomized, prospective double-blind placebo-controlled study. Int Endod J 2005;38(12):877-81.

2. Happonen RP, Bäckström AC, Ylipaavalniemi P. Prophylactic use of phenoxymethylpenicillin and tinidazole in mandibular third molar surgery, a comparative placebo controlled clinical trial. Br J Oral Maxillofac Surg 1990;28(1):12-5.

3. Hill M. No benefit from prophylactic antibiotics in third molar surgery. Evid Based Dent 2005;6(1):10.

4. Siddiqi A, Morkel JA, Zafar S. Antibiotic prophylaxis in third molar surgery: A randomized double-blind placebo-controlled clinical trial using split-mouth technique. Int J Oral Maxillofac Surg 2010;39(2):107-14.

5. Faculty of Dental Surgery. National Clinical Guidelines. London: The Royal College of Surgeons of England, 1997.

6. Flores MT, Andersson L, Andreasen JO, Bakland LK, Malmgren B, Barnett F, et al. Guidelines for the management of traumatic dental injuries. II. Avulsion of permanent teeth. Dent Traumatol 2007;23(3):130-6.

7. Herrera D, Alonso B, Leon R, Roldan S, Sanz M. Antimicrobial therapy in periodontitis: the use of systemic antimicrobials against the subgingival biofilm. J Clin Periodontol 2008;35(8 Suppl):45-66.

8. Pack PD, Haber J. The incidence of clinical infection after periodontal surgery. A retrospective study. J Periodontol 1983;54(7):441-3.

9. Abu-Ta'a M, Quirynen M, Teughels W, van Steenberghe D. Asepsis during periodontal surgery involving oral implants and the usefulness of peri-operative antibiotics: a prospective, randomized, controlled clinical trial. J Clin Periodontol 2008;35(1):58-63.

10. Esposito M, Grusovin MG, Coulthard P, Oliver R, Worthington HV. The efficacy of antibiotic prophylaxis at placement of dental implants: a Cochrane systematic review of randomised controlled clinical trials. Eur J Oral Implantol 2008;1(2):95-103.

11. Killey HC, Kay LW. An analysis of 250 cases of oro-antral fistula treated by the buccal flap operation. Oral Surg Oral Med Oral Pathol 1967;24(6):726-39.

12. Gould FK, Elliott TS, Foweraker J, Fulford M, Perry JD, Roberts GJ, et al. Guidelines for the prevention of endocarditis: report of the Working Party of the British Society for Antimicrobial Chemotherapy. J Antimicrob Chemother 2006;57(6):1035-42.

13. National Institute of Health and Clinical Excellence. CG64: Antimicrobial prophylaxis against infective endocarditis in adults and children undergoing interventional procedures. London: NICE; 2008. Available at: http://guidance.nice.org.uk/CG64. Accessed: Mar 2011.

14. Bartzokas CA, Johnson R, Jane M, Martin MV, Pearce PK, Saw Y. Relation between mouth and haematogenous infection in total joint replacements. Br Med J 1994;309(6953):506-8.

15. Berbari EF, Osmon DR, Carr A, Hanssen AD, Baddour LM, Greene D, et al. Dental Procedures as Risk Factors for Prosthetic Hip or Knee Infection: A Hospital-Based Prospective Case-Control Study. Clinical Infectious Diseases 2010;50(1):8-16.

16. Simmons NA, Ball AP, Cawson RA, Eykyn SJ, Hughes SP, McGowan DA, et al. Case against antibiotic prophylaxis for dental treatment of patients with joint prostheses [letter]. Lancet 1992;339(8788):301.

17. Little JW, Rhodus NL. The need for antibiotic prophylaxis of patients with penile implants during invasive dental procedures: a national survey of urologists. J Urol 1992;148(6):1801-4.

18. Joint Formulary Committee. British National Formulary. BNF 63 ed. London: British Medical Association and Royal Pharmaceutical Society of Great Britain; 2012. The reader is reminded that the BNF is constantly revised; for the latest guidelines please consult the current edition at www.BNF.org.

19. Lockhart PB, Loven B, Brennan MT, Fox PC. The evidence base for the efficacy of antibiotic prophylaxis in dental practice. J Am Dent Assoc 2007;138(4):458-74; quiz 534-5,

20. Edwards BJ, Hellstein JW, Jacobsen PL, Kaltman S, Mariotti A, Migliorati CA. Updated recommendations for managing the care of patients receiving oral bisphosphonate therapy: an advisory statement from the American Dental Association Council on Scientific Affairs. J Am Dent Assoc 2008;139:1674-1677.

21. Koga DH, Salvajoli JV, Alves FA. Dental extractions and radiotherapy in head and neck oncology: review of the literature. Oral Dis 2008;14(1):40-4.

12 ANTIVIRAL THERAPY

Viral infections are initially diagnosed on their clinical presentation and tend to be short-lived, but the orofacial tissues may be infected by several types of viruses. Infections with herpes simplex are common and can usually be managed in primary care with supportive therapy. Caution is necessary in patients who are severely immunocompromised or are unable to take fluids and at risk of dehydration. These patients should be referred to hospital. In addition, patients with prolonged infections which fail to resolve should be referred for further investigation.

Management of oral viral infections is symptomatic and usually involves:

- Rest.
- Plenty of fluids.
- Soft diet.
- Antipyretic analgesics.
- Antimicrobial mouthwash to reduce secondary infection. Chlorhexidine or hydrogen peroxide are suitable agents. The use of benzydamine mouthwash may provide some pain relief.

A small number of patients may require antivirals. Two nucleoside analogues are available for topical application: aciclovir and penciclovir. Aciclovir can also be given orally in suspension or tablet formulations.

12.1 Primary herpetic gingivostomatitis

This is caused by the herpes simplex virus, and most commonly presents in young children and young adults. The incubation period is approximately five days and infection can be subclinical. Management is primarily with supportive measures as outlined above. In severe cases, or if patients are immunocompromised, then systemic antiviral therapy is indicated.

ACICLOVIR

Adults

Aciclovir 200mg five times daily for five days[1,2]

Children

- 6 months-2 years: 100mg five times daily for five days
- 3-18 years: 200mg five times daily for five days

Available on prescription as:

- Aciclovir tablets 200mg
- Aciclovir oral suspension 200mg/5ml

If a patient fails to respond to therapy, they should be referred to a specialist to exclude underlying systemic conditions.

12.2 Secondary (recurrent) herpes simplex infections

Synonyms: herpes labialis, cold sores

Following a primary herpetic gingivostomatitis infection, herpes simplex remains latent in the trigeminal ganglion, and approximately one third of people develop herpes labialis and a secondary infection from reactivation of the virus.

The application of topical antiviral preparations has been found to reduce the progression of herpes labialis if it is applied early, ideally in the prodromal phase of the lesion.[3-5]

ACICLOVIR

Adults and children all ages
Apply cream to lesions every four hours (five times daily) for 5-10 days, starting at the first signs of infection

Available on prescription as aciclovir cream 5%

OR

PENICICLOVIR

Adults
Apply cream to lesions every two hours during waking hours for four days, starting at the first signs of infection

Children

- Under 12 years: not recommended
- 12 years and older: as for adults

Available on prescription as peniciclovir cream 1%

12.3 Orofacial herpes zoster infections

Synonyms: shingles, varicella

Systemic antivirals are advised in patients with herpes zoster infections as they have been found to reduce the incidence of the distressing complication of postherpetic neuralgia[6] and viral shedding. The reduction in viral shedding is beneficial as it can reduce the risk of corneal infection. Patients with herpes zoster affecting the first division of the trigeminal nerve with vesicles and/or ulceration involving the eye should be referred for an urgent ophthalmological opinion and treatment. Treatment with antivirals should be commenced as soon as possible and within 72 hours of the onset of the rash. Patients who are immunocompromised should be referred to a specialist medical practitioner.

ACICLOVIR

Adults

Aciclovir 800mg five times daily for seven days

Children

Not relevant for children in primary dental care setting; aciclovir is not licensed for the treatment of herpes zoster in children.

Available on prescription as:

- Aciclovir tablets 200mg
- Aciclovir tablets 800mg
- Aciclovir suspension 200mg/5ml

References

1. Nasser M, Fedorowicz Z, Khoshnevisan MH, Shahiri Tabarestani M. Acyclovir for treating primary herpetic gingivostomatitis. Cochrane Database Syst Rev 2008(4):CD006700.

2. Amir J, Harel L, Smetana Z, Varsano I. Treatment of herpes simplex gingivostomatitis with aciclovir in children: a randomised double blind placebo controlled study. B Med J 1997;314(7097):1800-3.

3. Worrall G. (2006) *Herpes labialis*. Clin Evidence. BMJ Publishing Group Ltd. http://www.clinicalevidence.com

4. Fiddian AP, Yeo JM, Stubbings R, Dean D. Successful treatment of herpes labialis with topical acyclovir. Br Med J (Clin Res Ed) 1983;286(6379):1699-701.

5. Femiano F, Gombos F, Scully C. Recurrent herpes labialis: efficacy of topical therapy with penciclovir compared with acyclovir (aciclovir). Oral Dis 2001;7(1):31-3.

6. Moomaw MD, Cornea P, Rathbun RC, Wendel KA. Review of antiviral therapy for herpes labialis, genital herpes and herpes zoster. Expert Rev Anti Infect Ther 2003;1(2):283-95.

13 ANTIFUNGAL THERAPY

Most oral fungal infections are caused by imperfect yeasts belonging to the genus Candida. Oral candidosis (candidiasis) is most notably associated with Candida albicans; however, a number of other Candida species are found as commensals in the oral mucosa and may be putative pathogens (eg. *C glabrata*, *C tropicalis*, *C krusei*).

A number of factors predispose to candidosis; these include antibiotic therapy, systemic and inhalation steroid therapy, immunosuppressive medication, anaemia, endocrine disorders including diabetes, salivary gland hypofunction, extremes of age and disorders of the immune system.

Immunodeficiencies have been highlighted as a cause of candidosis in HIV-positive individuals. When considering a differential diagnosis for persistent oral candidosis, HIV infection should be considered as a possible cause.

The clinician must always be mindful that oral candidosis may be a clinical marker for an underlying predisposing condition.

Several classifications of oral fungal infections have been used, but the most frequently adopted is the Samaranayake and MacFarlane classification.[1,2] This system divides the infection into primary oral candidosis (localised to oral and perioral tissues) and secondary oral candidosis (generalised candidal infections of mucosal membranes and cutaneous surfaces of the body). Mucocutaneous candidosis is mostly associated with patients who have primary immune deficiencies.

Clinically oral candidosis presents as three main variants: pseudomembranous, erythematous and hyperplastic.

13.1 Management of superficial infections

Superficial infections can be treated in a primary care setting; however, chronic hyperplastic candidosis is potentially premalignant, and patients should be referred to a specialist.

Local measures: When corticosteroid inhalers are thought to be causing or contributing to oral candidosis then the patient should be advised to rinse their mouth with water or clean their teeth immediately following the use of the inhaler.

Antifungal agents: The choice of topical antifungal agents has been drastically reduced with the withdrawal of amphotericin lozenges and nystatin pastilles. The only polyene antifungal that can now be prescribed is nystatin suspension. Miconazole, a topical imidazole agent, is available as an oromucosal gel, cream and as a combined preparation with hydrocortisone (ointment and cream). Fluconazole, a triazole antifungal agent, is available as an oral suspension and as capsules.

13.2 Pseudomembranous candidosis

Synonyms: thrush, pseudomembranous candidiasis

This condition is characterised by creamy white plaques, which can be dislodged to leave raw bleeding mucosa. These lesions can appear on any part of the oral mucosa and pharynx. This may be caused by inhaled corticosteroids, cytotoxic drugs, broad-spectrum antibiotics, or salivary gland hypofunction. However, pseudomembranous candidosis can be caused by underlying systemic conditions such as blood dyscrasias, malignancy, or immunosuppression.

Antifungal therapy of choice is nystatin suspension, miconazole or fluconazole. There is little difference in effectiveness.[3]

NYSTATIN

Adults

Nystatin 100,000 units four times daily after food for seven days, or continued for two days after lesions have healed. Advise patient to rinse the liquid around their mouth and then hold it against the lesions for five minutes, if possible, before swallowing.

Children

1 month-18 years: Use adult dose as above

Available on prescription as nystatin oral suspension 100,000 units/ml

OR

MICONAZOLE

Adults

Apply 5-10ml to the affected area four times daily after food. Use for seven days, or longer if required. Treatment should be continued for two days after lesions have healed.

Children

- 1 month-2 years: 2.5ml twice daily smeared around the mouth. Use for seven days, or longer if required. Treatment should be continued for two days after lesions have healed.

continued...

- 2 -6 years: 5ml twice daily after food. Use for seven days, or longer if required. Treatment should be continued for two days after lesions have healed.
- 6 -12 years: 5ml four times daily after food. Use for seven days, or longer if required. Treatment should be continued for two days after lesions have healed.
- 12-18 years: 5-10ml four times daily after food. Use for seven days, or longer if required. Treatment should be continued for two days after lesions have healed.

Available on prescription as miconazole oromucosal gel 24mg/ml

OR

FLUCONAZOLE

Adults

Fluconazole 50mg once daily for 7-14 days (maximum 14 days unless severely immunocompromised; these patients should be referred to a specialist or to a general medical practitioner)

Children

- 6 months-12 years: 3-6mg/kg on first day then 3mg/kg (max 100mg) daily for 7-14 days (maximum 14 days; see note for adults above)
- 12-18 years: 50mg once daily for 7-14 days (maximum 14 days; see note for adults above)

Available on prescription as:

- Fluconazole capsules 50mg
- Fluconazole oral suspension 50mg/5ml

If the patient does not respond to local measures and antifungal therapy, they should be referred for further investigation.

13.3 Erythematous candidosis

Synonyms: antibiotic sore mouth, acute atrophic candidosis

Erythematous candidosis may involve most areas of the oral mucosa and may be painful for the patient. It can be an acute or chronic condition, depending upon the duration of the condition. The condition can have similar predisposing factors to those seen in pseudomembranous candidosis. Typically it has been associated with broad-spectrum antibiotics or the use of steroid inhalers. The condition may result from pseudomembranous candidosis following loss of the pseudomembrane.

The treatment of erythematous candidosis is the same for pseudomembranous candidosis (see above). Local management of denture-related problems should be undertaken before antifungal therapy is commenced.

13.4 Chronic hyperplastic candidosis

Synonyms: hyperplastic candidiasis, candidal leukoplakia.

This chronic form of candidosis presents as a clearly defined, fixed, raised white patch that may be speckled or nodular. It can occur anywhere in the mouth, but has classically been associated with the commissures of the mouth.

This is generally considered to be a premalignant lesion and a biopsy is required. **The patient should be referred to a specialist.**

13.5 Chronic mucocutaneous candidosis

Patients with secondary oral candidosis such as in chronic mucocutaneous candidosis are identified and diagnosed early in life. They have immune defects or endocrinopathies. Hyperplastic plaque-like lesions are seen intra-orally and skin lesions are also visible. Nail defects (candidal paronychia) may be present. **Specialist advice is required for this group of patients.**

13.6 Candida-associated lesions

13.6.1 Chronic erythematous candidosis

Synonyms: denture stomatitis, denture sore mouth

This is usually characterised by inflammation on the denture-bearing maxillary mucosa. Predisposing factors should be eliminated before administering antifungal agents, but they are sometimes required as an adjunct to local measures before constructing new dentures.

Local measures:

- Strict denture hygiene using regular chemical and mechanical cleansing of dentures twice a day.
- Leave dentures out at night.
- Leave dentures out whenever it is feasible to do so during the day.
- Tissue conditioners/soft linings may be used to minimise mucosal trauma in poorly fitting dentures prior to construction of new dentures.

If the above measures are unsuccessful, new dentures should be made.

Antifungal therapy is as follows:

MICONAZOLE

Adults

Remove dentures and apply 5-10ml to the affected area four times daily, until 48 hours after the lesions resolve. The dentures can be reinserted to keep the gel in place.

continued...

Children

- 6-12 years old: apply 5ml to the affected area four times daily, until 48 hours after the lesions resolve. The dentures can be reinserted to keep the gel in place.
- 12-18 years : use adult dose

Available on prescription as miconazole oromucosal gel 24mg/ml

OR

FLUCONAZOLE

Adults

50mg once daily for 7-14 days (maximum 14 days unless severely immunocompromised; these patients should be referred to specialist or general medical practitioner).

Children

- 6 months-12 years: 3-6mg/kg on first day, then 3mg/kg (max 100mg) daily for 7- 14 days
- 12-18 years: 50mg once daily for 7-14 days (maximum 14 days; see note for adults above).

Available on prescription as:

- Fluconazole capsules 50mg
- Fluconazole oral suspension 50mg/5ml

13.6.2 Angular cheilitis (stomatitis)

This condition presents as cracking and inflammation of the angles of the mouth. It is commonly a candida-associated lesion. The condition is most frequently seen in patients who have denture-related stomatitis. However, as in other oral candidal infections it can be caused by underlying systemic disease such as deficiency anaemias, eating disorders, eczema, orofacial granulomatosis, Crohn's disease and immune deficiencies. An inadequate vertical face height is also a possible predisposing condition.

Angular cheilitis has a multifactorial aetiology and may be caused by a mixed candidal-bacterial infection. In patients who do not wear dentures, bacterial infections with staphylococci and/or streptococci are more likely to be cultured from the lesions.

Predisposing factors should be managed (eg. resolution of intraoral reservoir of candida in patients with chronic erythematous candidosis, new dentures). Miconazole cream should be the first choice anti-infective agent as it has antifungal activity and some activity against gram-positive cocci.

In cases that are proven to be staphylococci, sodium fusidate ointment is indicated. When the lesions are unresponsive, it may be worth trying a combination of miconazole with hydrocortisone. Refractory cases should be referred for specialist opinion.

When angular cheilitis is associated with chronic erythematous candidosis, the intraoral infection should be treated concomitantly to eliminate the palatal reservoir.

MICONAZOLE

Adults and children

Apply to angles of the mouth twice daily for 10 days or until lesions have healed

Available on prescription as miconazole cream

OR

SODIUM FUSIDATE

Adults and children

Apply to angles of the mouth three to four times daily for no longer than 10 days

Available on prescription as sodium fusidate ointment

OR

MICONAZOLE AND HYDROCORTISONE

Adults and children

Apply to angles of the mouth twice a day for a maximum of seven days

Available on prescription as:

- Miconazole and hydrocortisone cream
- Miconazole and hydrocortisone ointment

Note that creams are used on wet surfaces and ointments on dry surfaces

13.6.3 Median rhomboid glossitis (glossal central papillary atrophy)

This condition is uncommon. and consists of a well demarcated area of depapillation on the midline of the dorsum of the tongue (just anterior to the circumvallate papillae). It may be associated with candida.

Predisposing factors include smoking, denture-wearing, corticosteroid sprays and HIV. Predisposing factors should be removed and antifungal therapy initiated, as it can sometimes be successful at reducing or resolving the lesion.

Systemic fluconazole appears to be more successful than topical agents. However, patients with a provisional diagnosis of median rhomboid glossitis should have blood tests to exclude haematinic deficiencies. Very occasionally, a biopsy may be indicated.

References

1. Macfarlane TW, Samaranayake LP. Oral candidosis. London: Butterworth-Heinemann; 1990.

2. Axell T, Samaranayake LP, Reichart PA, Olsen I. A proposal for reclassification of oral candidosis. Oral Surg Oral Med Oral Pathol Oral Radiol Endod 1997;84(2):111-2.

3. Blomgren J, Berggren U, Jontell M. Fluconazole versus nystatin in the treatment of oral candidosis. Acta Odontol Scand 1998;56(4):202-5.